Live to be 120, die healthily:

New Scientific Data Suggest Faith in God Can Prolong Life

World Under God's Judgment

Messenger K. Hezekiah Scipio

Copyright © 2015, K. Hezekiah Scipio

Published by Biblical Health Center Inc. Nonprofit
Tax exempted under 501(c)3 Internal Revenue Code.
Founder: Messenger K. Hezekiah Scipio

P.O.Box 291964
Tampa, Fl 33687

Email : biblicalhealthcenter@gmail.com
www.biblicalhealthcenter.com
www.biblicalhealthcenter.net
www.biblicalhealthcenter.org
http://www.godsplantthatheal.org/

Acknowledgment

The Lord placed this message on my heart since 2008, but I lacked the courage to proclaim it because I did not know whether I was merely wishful-thinking or that I was indeed, responding to the prompting of the Holy Spirit. Furthermore, I did not trust that my writing skill measured up well enough.

Then, Jehovah God Almighty performed a miracle in my life, showing me that he is God, and he can prolong life; I was 100 years of age (take away twenty-five years) when Jehovah sent his Angel in the person of Mary Roberts, Students' Primary Advisor at Siena Heights University, College of Professional Studies, Adrian, Michigan, through the National Certification Board for Therapeutic Massage and Bodywork (NCBTMB) to let me know that SHU was granting me admission to its bachelor's degree program in Applied Science.

At Siena Heights University, I was privileged to meet among its faculty members, three wonderful Professors : Professor Anthony Farina, Professor Gail A. Ryder, and Dr. Parvindar Mehta who became my instant guides, and began bringing me out of my insecurities about grammar, punctuations, research, and everything else. I cannot thank them well enough. I am also thankful to Tracy Jones of NCBTMB, my brother and sister Pastor Nestor Konan, and Pastor Patricia Byrd-Konan for their encouragements, and to my fellow classmates, especially Michael Mull, Marisa Moore , Charneal Kitchen, and Donna

Riley, whose suggestions, comments, and corrections were reassurances of the rightness of this message. As far as I am concerned, these wonderful people are Angels that God placed on my path. Thank you all. . – K. Hezekiah Scipio

"In the path of righteousness there is life,

in walking its path there is no death."

Proverbs 12:28

The Watchman's Duty

1 Again the word of the LORD came unto me, saying,
2 Son of man, speak to the children of thy people, and say unto them, When I bring the sword upon a land, if the people of the land take a man of their coasts, and set him for their watchman:
3 if when he seeth the sword come upon the land, he blow the trumpet, and warn the people;
4 then whosoever heareth the sound of the trumpet, and taketh not warning; if the sword come, and take him away, his blood shall be upon his own head.
5 He heard the sound of the trumpet, and took not warning; his blood shall be upon him. But he that taketh warning shall deliver his soul.
6 But if the watchman see the sword come, and blow not the trumpet, and the people be not warned; if the sword come, and take *any* person from among them, he is taken away in his iniquity; but his blood will I require at the watchman's hand.
7 ¶ So thou, O son of man, I have set thee a watchman unto the house of Israel; therefore thou shalt hear the word at my mouth, and warn them from me.
8 When I say unto the wicked, O wicked *man,* thou shalt surely die; if thou dost not speak to warn the wicked from his way, that wicked *man* shall die in his

iniquity; but his blood will I require at thine hand.

9 Nevertheless, if thou warn the wicked of his way to turn from it; if he do not turn from his way, he shall die in his iniquity; but thou hast delivered thy soul. **(Ezekiel 33:1-9)**

Psalm 15

1. Jehovah, who shall sojourn in your tabernacle? Who shall dwell in your holy mountain?

2. He that walks in integrity, and who does justice, and speaks the truth in his heart;

3. Who slanders not with his tongue, who does no evil to his fellow, nor takes up a reproach against his neighbor;

4. In whose eyes the vile person is condemned, but who honors them that fear Jehovah; who, when he swears to his fellow, changes not;

5. Who puts not out his money to usury, nor takes a bribe against the innocent, He that does these things shall never be moved.

The Internal Sense

That they who love their neighbor and God, will be of the Lord's church, verses 1—5

Join THE BODY OF CHRIST
at
BIBLICAL HEALTH CENTER INC.,

•a nonprofit organization in Tampa, Florida, tax exempted under 501(c)3 of the Internal Revenue Code

•**Email : biblicalhealthcenter@gmail.com**

Apostle Paul sums up our purpose this way:

"For to me, to live is Christ, and to die is gain." (Philippians 1 : 21)

•We proclaim the gospel of Our Lord Jesus Christ, worship Jehovah God Almighty, pray, practise biblical meditation, biblical massage, sing hymns, observe strict micro nutrient dietary regimen as therapy for improved health and longevity , and for healing the Spirit, mind and body.

There is no distance too far away from Almighty God. "For where two or three gather in my name, there am I with them." (Matthews 18:20) **Email us. Let**

us get together in the Spirit while praying for a
renewed life in Christ Jesus. Amen .

Proverbs 8 (KJV)

Doth not wisdom cry? and understanding put forth her voice?

2 She standeth in the top of high places, by the way in the places of the paths.

3 She crieth at the gates, at the entry of the city, at the coming in at the doors.

4 Unto you, O men, I call; and my voice is to the sons of man.

5 O ye simple, understand wisdom: and, ye fools, be ye of an understanding heart.

6 Hear; for I will speak of excellent things; and the opening of my lips shall be right things.

7 For my mouth shall speak truth; and wickedness is an abomination to my lips.

8 All the words of my mouth are in righteousness; there is nothing froward or perverse in them.

9 They are all plain to him that understandeth, and right to them that find knowledge.

10 Receive my instruction, and not silver; and knowledge rather than choice gold.

11 For wisdom is better than rubies; and all the things that may be desired are not to be compared to it.

12 I wisdom dwell with prudence, and find out knowledge of witty inventions.

13 The fear of the Lord is to hate evil: pride, and arrogancy, and the evil way, and the froward mouth, do I hate.

14 Counsel is mine, and sound wisdom: I am understanding; I have strength.

15 By me kings reign, and princes decree justice.

16 By me princes rule, and nobles, even all the judges of the earth.

17 I love them that love me; and those that seek me early shall find me.

18 Riches and honour are with me; yea, durable riches and righteousness.

19 My fruit is better than gold, yea, than fine gold; and my revenue than choice silver.

20 I lead in the way of righteousness, in the midst of the paths of judgment:

21 That I may cause those that love me to inherit substance; and I will fill their treasures.

22 The Lord possessed me in the beginning of his way, before his works of old.

23 I was set up from everlasting, from the beginning, or ever the earth was.

24 When there were no depths, I was brought forth; when there were no fountains abounding with water.

25 Before the mountains were settled, before the hills was I brought forth:

26 While as yet he had not made the earth, nor the fields, nor the highest part of the dust of the world.

27 When he prepared the heavens, I was there: when he set a compass upon the face of the depth:

28 When he established the clouds above: when he strengthened the fountains of the deep:

29 When he gave to the sea his decree, that the waters should not pass his commandment: when he appointed the foundations of the earth:

30 Then I was by him, as one brought up with him: and I was daily his delight, rejoicing always before him;

31 Rejoicing in the habitable part of his earth; and my delights were with the sons of men.

32 Now therefore hearken unto me, O ye children: for blessed are they that keep my ways.

33 Hear instruction, and be wise, and refuse it not.

34 Blessed is the man that heareth me, watching daily at my gates, waiting at the posts of my doors.

35 For whoso findeth me findeth life, and shall obtain favour of the Lord.

36 But he that sinneth against me wrongeth his own soul: all they that hate me love death

"It's a warning...a wake up call.""

"Those who despise the word bring destruction on themselves,

but those who respect the commandment will be rewarded." Proverbs 13:13

JUDGMENT. STOP !

"For it is time for judgment to begin with Jehovah God's household; and if it begins with us, what will the outcome be for those who do not obey the gospel of Jehovah?"   1 Peter 4:17

Turn away from evil. The world is under God's fierce judgment. There is evil in the churches; daylight robbery and syncretism abound. Syncretism is an abomination to the Lord, and yet Christians are practising yoga, tai chi, transcendental meditation, and ayurveda –   offshoots of Hinduism, Buddhism and Shintoism – idolatry .

God said , "I am Yahweh ; that is my name! I will not yield my glory to another or my praise to idols." (Isaiah 42:8)

Christians are doing what they please, and disobeying Almighty God. Evil goes on in high places of government; duplicity, hypocrisy and hatred hold sway among political leaders. Dishonesty and chicanery reign over business and financial worlds. There is no one to trust . Love turns into falsehood as wives turn against husbands, and children against their parents. God's anger is inflamed, people!Turn away from evil. The world is under God's judgment, don't you see?

God said, "Those who love me , I will deliver; I will protect those who know my name, when they call I will answer them; I will be with them in trouble, I will rescue them and honor them. With long life I will satisfy them and show them my salvation." (Psalm 91:14 -16)

Why are there so many people asking, "Are these signs of the End Times ? " Our Lord Jesus Christ warned in Matthew 24: 6-8,

> You are going to hear the noise of battles far away; but do not be troubled. Such things must happen, but they do not mean that the end has come. Countries will fight each other; kingdoms will attack one another. There will be famines and earthquakes everywhere. All these things are like the first pains of childbirth.

But these manifestations in our time are prophecies of Isaiah 65:1-23 in which Jehovah Almighty God warned he would judge the world for disobedience and reward obedience with longevity. Believers who trust Jehovah can happily look forward to living their full Genesis 6:3 lifespan of 120 years. These are not claims or assumptions based on blind faith ; scientific data prove that faith in God can prolong life. Isaiah predicted believers will

> live out their lifespan, and those who live to be a hundred will be considered young. To die before

that would be considered that I (Jehovah) had punished them. (Isaiah 65:20)

Some people believe that the age of 70 is the limit to life expectancy because a verse in the bible states that, "The days of our life are seventy years, or perhaps eighty, if we are strong; even then their span is only toil and trouble" (Psalm 90:10).

Some bible students dispute the claim; instead, they assert that Moses merely expressed his observation of people's lives. Still others point to another verse in the bible which states that "the Lord said, 'I will not allow people to live forever; they are mortal. From now on, they will live no longer than 120 years. (Genesis 6: 3, TEV)

Yet, others contend that none of those two interpretations is right. And yet, there are ample evidences in our plain sight that God has put in place for those who believe in his Son our Lord Jesus Christ ways that they can " reverse disease, reduce high blood pressure, lose weight, prevent heart attacks, improve health, and live a long life." (Joel Fuhrman, M.D, 2007)

For new scientific data suggest faith in God can prolong life, and experts say the first person to live to be 150 years old has already been born. We can see it with our own eyes, and can bear witnesses for ourselves that more people are living longer nowadays than ever before.

Some people attribute the reason to advances in medical science and technology, but if one looks around, one also sees on-going worldwide destruction ; millions of people are dying from wars, natural disasters, sickness and diseases, and people are killing one another out of hatred , racism, nationalism, or sheer greed. Wives are turning against their husbands, and sons and daughters against their fathers and mothers. Frightfully unusual things are happening all over the world: airplanes are disappearing from the sky , and the earth is suddenly giving way , and swallowing up anything standing on its way.

The good news is that Christians have no cause for concern because the world is witnessing the fulfillment of God's promise, and medical science is just catching up with Scripture in acknowledging that God is at work. Jehovah Almighty God promised

No more shall there be an infant...that lives but a few days , or an old person who does not live out a lifetime; for one who dies at a hundred years will be considered a youth, and one who falls short of a hundred will be considered accursed. They shall build houses and inhabit them; they shall plant vineyards and eat their fruit. They shall not build and another inhabit; they shall not plant and another eat; for like the days of a tree, shall the days of my people be, and my chosen shall long enjoy the work of their hands. They shall not labor in vain, or bear children for calamity; for they shall be offspring blessed by the Lord – and their descendants as well. (Isaiah 65:20-23)

What would you do if you had scientifically proven formula for living disease - free to be 120 years and in good health? You do not need any scientifically proven formula because Jehovah has already provided the formula in his Son Jesus , who spelled it all out for us many times over: "If you love me, obey my commandments." (John 14:15) "When you obey my commandments, you remain in my love, just as I obey my Father's commandments and remain in his love" (John 15:10)

Scientific Literature Supports It

Scientific literature claims that in merely 50 years from 2014, Americans will begin living to be very healthy and youthful at 100 years' age, and there are babies already born that will live to be 150 years old. (Barbara Walters, 2013)

Given the prediction by science that in just 50 years from 2014, Americans will live to be 100 years, the question is: what will people do to be 120 ? Can faith in God prolong life? What would you do if you had scientifically proven formula for living disease - free to be 120 years and not look old?

These predictions are not mere speculations. The indicators are showing that in the very near future human life will extend beyond 70 years as it was before the floods of Noah. In the ancient biblical world, people lived longer. Life expectancy began declining after the flood.

Change began manifesting over the last 2000 years showing a slow increase in life expectancy. Now scientists predict people will be able to live healthily into their 120th birthday; their skin will not wrinkle nor their hair turn gray, neither will their eyesight become weak nor will they lose their strength.

The most convincing forecast is a report in the New England Journal of Medicine (2005) predicting that by 2060, Americans and people in the developed world will live to be 100 years of age. In 2013, researchers at Pew Research Center Religion & Public Life Project made a more ambitious prediction following a study; people interviewed believed Americans would live to be 120 years in 37 years from 2013, not in 50 years as New England Journal of Medicine researchers predicted.

The causes of increase in life expectancy are advances in health care, childcare, seniors care, and nutrition care. There are fewer deaths in the delivery rooms nowadays than before, and older people are living much longer. Scientists, not only in America, but in Singapore, Russia, and China, have identified a variety of factors that will help prolong human life. These include new drugs that resourceful manufacturers are developing to boost "telomeres," in our body ; lack of "telomere enzymes" (Langmore, 2014) causes our body to age and die and so we die.

GOD IS RAISING THE DEAD

Science laboratories are also discovering new evidences suggesting adherence to biblical injunctions and practices will do just as much as telomerase supplements . The scientific data suggest that Jehovah heals !

Six thousand biblical years since creation, Jehovah God has told his people "I am the God that heals you." When a miracle occurs, and a sick person who is not expected to live, suddenly takes a surprising turn for the better and recovers, Christians, and their fellow believers give God the glory, saying "Jesus healed the person." The healthcare profession calls that phenomenon "spontaneous remission." (Lissa Rankin,2013)

When a person thinks an evil thought and it happens, Christians call it "demonic attack." The healthcare profession labels that experience "nocebo effect." (Rankin, 2013) When an ailing believer recovers from an illness following corporate or intercessory prayers, fellow believers give Jehovah God or Jesus Christ the glory for that person's recovery. Doctors say, it is "placebo effect." (Rankin, 2013)

Doctors stick to the teaching of medical textbooks and attribute healing to " the human body's innate ability to heal itself" (Herbert Benson, 2014) even though the human body did not create itself, and when the human body dies, it is D-E-A-D, and the dead has no innate ability to will itself to recovery.

There are numerous examples in our present day of people certified dead who suddenly came back to life: On Christmas Day 2009, according to CNN, a husband took his pregnant wife in labor to the delivery room. She had complications,and died together with her baby. Hours later, medical personnel saw life coming back into the baby, and next , the mother. Both mother and baby came back to life. They lived. Christians credited Jesus for their miraculous recovery but the medical profession claimed it was "spontaneous remission."

In West Virginia, U.S., on May 24, 2013, Velma Thomas was declared clinically brain dead for 17 hours after she had a heart attack in her home. She was placed on life support at the local Charleston Area Medical Center while doctors battled to bring her back to life. After her heart stopped three times and she had no detectable brain activity, doctors believed she would not survive, and thus, told family members and friends to begin planning a funeral.
"There were really no signs that she had neurological functions," Kevin Eggleston, an internal medicine

specialist, told ABC News.

After 10 minutes , her life support was turned off, while nurses were removing the tubing from the ventilator, suddenly Velma moved her arm, coughed and asked for her son, Tim Thomas. Velma lives again! Christians credited the hand of Jehovah God at work in her recovery but the medical profession gave the credit to "spontaneous remission." (Rankin, 2013)

In Missouri City, Texas, Erica Nigrelli, an English teacher at Elkins High School , was 36 weeks into her pregnancy when she started feeling faint, one February morning , NBC local affiliate KPRC reported. Nigrelli's desperate husband , a fellow teacher, called 911. Meanwhile, coworkers, Jennifer Longoria, June Tomlin and Maxine Reeves started doing CPR and located a nearby defibrillator to try to restart the pregnant woman's heart. At the hospital, doctors stopped CPR so that Elayna could be delivered by emergency cesarean section, "The doctors told me that Erica delivered postmortem because she did not have a heartbeat when they took the baby out," Nathan Nigrelli told The Star. (2013, May 23, Fort Bend Star) A miracle happened; life came back into the dead woman. Both mother and child live.

God works miracles. The miracle of healing is one of Jehovah's ways by which he glorifies himself. "Nothing is more certain than the fact that Jesus was a healer," writes, Dr. John Chirban, Director of the

Institute of Medicine , Psychology and Religion in Cambridge, Massachusetts at Harvard Medical School and the Cambridge Hospital. Chirban is among a growing number of healthcare authorities that acknowledge Jehovah God as healer of the sick.

"I AM The God that Heals You"

This growing school of practising physicians and healthcare professionals believe that patients are best served when therapy is directed at not only the physiological symptoms but emotional and Spiritual conditions as well. It prompted primary care provider and author, Dr. Christopher Hobbs to declare ; "As a primary care provider , I see many patients who aren't well served by today's modern healthcare system – people who are often encouraged to depend on drugs and medical procedure to fix symptoms and conditions without any mention of the personal power they possess to create and maintain health." (Hobbs, 1985)

Dr. Lissa Rankin, researcher, and author asserts, "Some combination of positive belief and the element of nurturing care of right healers can help turn off stress responses and activate the body's natural self repair systems in your body," and Dr. Erik Dalton (2005) , manual therapist, and researcher, rejoins, "Treatment results are always faster and better in those who maintain the feeling that they will improve. Defeatist attitude are signs that the client may not really want to improve." Dr. Mike Stangherlin (2009)   argues that "over the-counter and prescription painkillers do nothing to restore health; they actually harm several organ systems in the body."

At Rush University Medical Center, Chicago, researchers concluded that "a belief in a concerned GOD" (Murphy, 2010) is critical to good health and longevity. Following an eight-week study involving 136 adults suffering mental illnesses like depression and bipolar depression, investigators found that those with strong beliefs in a personal and concerned God were more likely to experience an improvement, according to Patricia Murphy, PhD, chaplain and an assistant professor of religion, health and human values at Rush University.

Murphy (2010) noted that, "the positive response to medication had little to do with the feeling of hope that typically accompanies spiritual belief," adding. "It was tied specifically to the belief that a Supreme Being cared."

In a related study, ScienceDaily website, citing the Journal of Affective Disorders, reported conclusions of studies in which researchers matched over a period of one year, the recovery expectation levels of 159 patients at McLean Hospital who believed in God, against those who had little or no belief.

According to David H. Rosmarin, PhD, McLean Hospital clinician and instructor in the Department of Psychiatry at Harvard Medical School, patients who expressed their faith in God, and an expectation of divine intervention in their recovery, experienced a much shorter time of healing than the patients who did not believe in God.

Rosmarin (2013) added that, "given the prevalence of religious belief in the United States -- over 90% of the population -- these findings are important in that they highlight the clinical implications of spiritual life."

Similar studies at the National Institutes of Health Center for Complementary and Alternative Medicine, concluded, "church attendance is correlated with increased longevity, or better health," Harvard professor, Anne Harrington, leading a team of researchers announced at the NIH Continuing Education workshop. Harrington (2013) noted that over the last ten years, increasing public interest in the effect of spirituality on health, spurred 70 of America's 125 leading medical schools to open research centers where medical students also study "spirituality's health connections." (Harrington, 2013)

In a related development , August 2013, researcher, Dr. Lissa Rankin, announced that scientific data proved that drugs do not cure diseases; instead, "some combination of positive belief and the nurturing care" of a trusted healthcare practitioner are critical to "activating the body's self-repair mechanism." (Rankin, 2013) The researcher added,

In order to be optimally healthy you need a healthy spiritual connection, a healthy relationship with neighbors, a healthy mind, a healthy environment, and a healthy money. You can pray or attend religious services. You may not think that your spiritual life or your relationships, or financial life affect the health of your body, but the scientific evidence proves that they do. (Rankin, 2013)

This study aligns with other independent separate studies by the American Society for Personality and Social Psychology (Pappas, 2013), and the American Institute of Stress (2014). Both institutions' researchers arrived at similar findings linking stress and loneliness with depression, anxiety, heart attacks, stroke, hypertension, and a host of numerous viral, emotional and physical disorders. Some research scientists therefore, urge medical professionals to exercise new treatment protocols which encourage patients' involvement in activities that draw on their spiritual convictions. A leading voice is Harvard professor emeritus at Harvard Medical School, Herbert Benson, M.D (2014).

The researcher claims (biblical) meditation can slow down the body's metabolism and reduce aging. Benson (2014) and his team found that an individual's spiritual persuasion was critical to the physiological effects of meditation. The scientist asserts,

> Meditation based on affirmative beliefs…brought forth remembered wellness. Reviving top down, nerve cell firing patterns in the brain that were associated with wellness. When present, faith in an eternal or life transcending force seemed to make the fullest use of remembered wellness because it is a supremely soothing belief, disconnecting unhealthy logic and worries. (Benson, 2014)

It is significant that the bible relates the benefits of biblical meditation and fasting, and provides guidelines for them: God commanded,

> This book of the law shall not depart out of your mouth. You shall meditate on it day and night, so that you may be careful to act in accordance with all that is written in it. For then you shall make your way prosperous, and then you shall be successful. (Joshua 1:8)

Further, into the scripture, are instructions on how a meditative individual should focus his or her thoughts to obtain "the peace of God which passes all understanding."(Philippians 4:7). Benson (2014) refers to this state of mind as the "relaxation response."

The National Institutes of Health Center for
Complementary and Alternative Medicine researcher
physician Joel Fuhrman suggests adding "supervised
therapeutic fasting" to the treatment menu, arguing that
, "therapeutic fasting accelerates the healing process and
allows the body to recover from serious disease in a
dramatically short period of time." Fuhrman writes,

> In my practice I have seen fasting eliminate lupus
> and arthritis, remove chronic skin conditions such
> as psoriasis and eczema, health the digestive tract
> in patients with ulcerative colitis and Crohn's
> disease, and quickly eliminate cardiovascular
> diseases such as high blood pressure and angina.
> In these cases the recoveries were permanent:
> fasting enabled longtime disease sufferers
> unchain themselves from their multiple toxic
> dugs and even eliminate the need for surgery,
> which was recommended to some of them as their
> only solution.(Fuhrman, 2005)

Isaiah 58 records Jehovah God's guidelines for
fasting, and its benefits, with Jehovah promising that,
"If you honor it, not going your own ways, serving your
own interest, or pursuing your own affairs; then you
shall take delight in the LORD, and I will make you ride
upon the heights of the earth" (Isaiah 58:13-14)

FAITH IN GOD PART OF MEDICAL MENU

Healing through faith in Jehovah God and his Son Jesus Christ, once activity confined to churches and "faith healers," is becoming part of the medical establishment's prescription for illnesses (Harrington, 2013). One powerful medical prescription from scripture for improved health and longevity is a person's ability to forgive past transgressions.

In a ten-year study , Dr. Everett Worthington, Professor of Psychology at Virginia Commonwealth University and a team of researchers concluded that , "unforgiveness toward a transgressor is linked to a variety of health issues and can be a deadly virus if left untreated." (Worthington, 1990)

At Hope College in Holland, Michigan, investigators asked cohorts, while testing their heart rates, sweat emissions and other responses, to remember past wrongs. "Their blood pressure increases, their heart rate increases, and their muscle tensions are also higher, suggesting their stress responses are greater during their unforgiving than forgiving conditions." (Witvliet, 2001)

This demonstration of positive or negative effects of unforgiveness tie in with the teachings of our Lord

Jesus Christ; he taught that, "When you do not forgive transgressions against you, your Father in heaven will not forgive you." (Mark 11:26)

Scientific data show that unforgiveness impedes spiritual, emotional and physical healing. It floods the unforgiving person's internal system with cortisol and epinephrine, poisonous hormones causing him or her to fall sick (Worthington, 1990). If the person is already sick, he or she does not easily heal. The one who quickly forgives past wrongs is also the person who heals quickly, and is more likely to live a longer life.

Based on these data, it is safe to suggest the target of 120 years' life expectancy is not a farfetched daydream; it is attainable if people observe some specific principles, which include prayer, biblical meditation, constant study and application of Scripture, and maintaining regular micro-nutrient dietary regimen, with daily exercise.

Paralleling this hope of longevity however, is the fear that people may start thinking they are gods, ignoring the complexity of life as they manufacture and take immortality drugs resulting in provoking God's anger and in turn invoking upon the world the worst kind of the "tower of babel."(Genesis 11:1-9)

It is better to believe in Jesus Christ and live by his teachings, in particular, "The Greatest Commandment" ; it is key to longevity and salvation. In the Greatest Commandment, Jesus taught , "You must love the Lord your God with all your heart, and with all your mind and with all your soul; you must love your neighbor as yourself, "(Matthew 22:37-40).

If anyone will love God, "with all the heart, and with all the soul, and with all the mind…and to love a neighbor as self" (Matthew 22:37-40), that individual must care for his or her own body as well; sexual immorality and idolatry are as poisonous to the body as smoking, drunkenness and drug addiction. The person must treat the body as "the temple of the Holy Spirit." When the individual sees himself or herself as pure, he or she will treat his or her neighbor as pure – as image of God . Titus 1:15 reminds us, "To the pure, all things are pure, but to those who are corrupted and do not believe, nothing is pure. In fact, both their minds and consciences are corrupted". So it is fitting that people feed their bodies with the nutrient specific to each of the three components of the body, namely, the Spirit, soul and body.

Just as the Spirit and the Soul need their own spiritual food, the physical body needs its own specific foods to keep it functioning. A person who "loves God with all the heart and with all the mind and with all the soul", and loves his neighbor, will faithfully observe God's instructions on the things to eat and not to eat, and note that "plants will be for food…and for healing." (Ezekiel 47:12)

PLANTS, FOR FOOD...AND HEALING

Nutrition researchers note that there are conclusive evidences that eating micro-nutrient diet will prevent, or reverse disease, improve health, and prolong a disease-free life. These scientists believe that eating "micro-nutrient rich" meals can "reduce asthma, ear infections, and allergies, and protect children for the future against diabetes, cardiovascular disease and cancer," (Fuhrman, 2005).

They argue that eating micro-nutrient meals is integral to the protocol for healthy living or longevity. Adhering to micro-nutrient dietary practice will help restore diminished building blocks for improved health and longevity. Dr. Fuhrman (2005), a leading researcher with the National Institutes of Health Center for Complementary and Alternative   Medicine, blames the types of foods most people ate in their formative years as "the primary cause of disease and premature death." (Fuhrman, 2005)

The researcher asserts, "We can't smoke with impunity, excessively consume alcohol without paying a price, or eat the typical American diet and not eventually develop atherosclerotic heart disease and cancer." (Fuhrman, 2005)

As the types of foods that people ate in infancy affect their health and growth into adulthood, it will help if mothers feed their babies foods that enhance their children's growth. Feeding children micro-nutrient based foods while bringing them up in the fear and admonition of the Lord will ensure the children's longevity even as their Spiritual salvation is assured. Advocates of micro-nutrient rich dietary practice assert that the biblical injunction in Proverbs 22:6, "train up a child in the way he should go: and when he is old, he will not depart from it," applies as well to the foods parents feed their children. Fuhrman (2005) advises new mothers feed their babies on milk from their own breasts and never on a diet centered on animal's milk.

Parents should avoid eating meat, cheese, butter, pasta, and white bread, salt, caffeine, sugar filled snacks and drinks, because those foods are poison; they lay the groundwork for cancer, diabetes, and heart disease. New mothers should not feed their children foods that will inadvertently cause their children to develop later on in life autoimmune illnesses . Parents and their children should keep away from white-colored foods. For better health and longevity, it is good to eat fresh foods, vegetables, beans, raw nuts and seeds, brussels sprouts, broccoli sprouts, kale, berries, grapes, black berries, blue berries, fruits, and turmeric roots. (Fuhrman, 2005)

SCRIPTURE

Scripture instructs that the body is a temple of the Holy Spirit. (1 Corinthians 6:19) It is important that a person does not defile the body with foods that are toxic; it is equally important that a person must not indulge in activities that spiritually corrupt the body.

Restricting one's self to micro-nutrient diet although not a requirement for salvation or spiritual development, it is nonetheless a discipline that can help a person to structure his or her own spiritual life. The belief that eating micronutrient rich diet helps in restoring diminished building blocks for improved health and longevity, spurred studies at Loma Linda University Medical Center, California (Adventists Health Studies ,n.d).

The studies show that God-believing vegan and vegetarian Seventh Day Adventists, live ten to fifteen years longer than do most Americans. The study considered lifestyles, diet, and belief as significant factors.

Studies, conducted over twelve years of more than 30,000 cohorts, showed that the participants who were over 83 years of age, and who consumed nuts at least five times a week, "had 39% lower risk of death by Coronary Heart Disease. Younger people who ate nuts five times every week, had 48 percent lower risk of death by CHD than those who ate nuts less than once every week" (Higdon & Drake, 2007).

Scientists put together information from five studies, comparing "death rates from common diseases of 76,172 men and women vegetarians, ages 16-89 with non-vegetarians of similar lifestyles and ages. Vegetarians did not eat meat or fish. The death rate from heart attack was lower among the vegetarians than those who were no vegetarians. The death rate by heart attack among regular meat eaters was higher than those who were occasional meat eaters, and lower by 34% among those who ate fish and not meat.

Similar investigations are on-going involving 96.000 Seventh Day Adventists of Canada and America to find out connections, if there are any, between religion, lifestyles, diet and diseases. (Adventists Health Studies, n.d).

What do Americans think or say about living to be 120 years and beyond? The investigation found that Americans feared that longevity would prolong sufferings through sickness and diseases. (Saletan, 2013) For beauty conscious Americans, the thought of becoming wrinkled up, and sick, with accompanying diseases of gerontology, made death a more welcoming prospect. Research continues in "the universities and corporate laboratories aiming at unlocking the secrets of aging while religious leaders, bioethicists and philosophers consider the morality of radical life extension" (Pew Research Religion and Public Life Project, 2013).

Pew Research Center surveyed 2000 people to find out if Americans would agree to a bio-genetic procedure to slow down their growth hormones enabling them live to be 120; about 56% of those interviewed said "no." Although all of those interviewed believed that in 36 years, that is, by 2050, people will begin living to be 120 years, most did not want to have anything to do with biological or genetically engineering of their bodies in order to live that long. (Saletan, 2013)

ACCEPT JESUS CHRIST AS YOUR SAVIOR

Many people believe that the best solution is to go back and live as Jesus Christ taught,so that if the believer should die regardless of the age, he or she will be expected to live , fulfilling the promise of our Lord Jesus, "...he who believes in me will live even if he dies, and everyone who lives and believes in me will never die. "(John 11:25-26)

Our Lord Jesus taught in Matthew 22:37-40, "Love God with all your heart, and with all your soul, and with all your mind; and love your neighbor as yourself." This is central to his teaching , and it is the seed for peace and longevity. For God created human beings to be gregarious."The Lord said, 'It is not good for the man to be alone.'" (Genesis 2:18) Love of a neighbor alleviates loneliness.

A study by the Society for Personality and Social Psychology revealed that lonely people are prone to stress, a factor implicated in heart disorders, according to Pappas (2013). "You may not think that your spiritual life or your relationships, or financial life affect the health of your body, but the scientific evidence proves that they do" (Rankin, 2013).

Why or how do human beings age, and die? The question prompted the interest for scientific studies by a team of biologists under the leadership of Dr. John Langmore (2014), at Michigan University's Department of Biology. Researchers believed that human beings would have the potential to live forever someday if scientists could identify the agents of aging to enable resourceful manufacturers produce an antidote; surprisingly, researchers have identified in the human body, certain cells that link with the production of cancer and aging. The cells are called "telomeres enzymes." (Langmore, 2014) They are like protective caps at the end of our genetic code. As our body grows, the cells in the body outgrow the telomeres rendering the telomeres shorter and shorter and causing the body to age and die; but stress, smoking, obesity, lack of exercise and a poor diet can also cause telomeres to shrink and cause human cells to age and die. Our genetic code need telomeres' protection, for our bodies to endure.

Since shorter telomeres cause the body to age quickly ,and a woman's bones and mineral density to decrease fast, lengthening telomeres will result in renewing a person's DNA and prolonging his or her life in perpetuity.

Scientists are therefore, working on developing "telomerase" supplements enabling human beings to renew their genetic code and prolong their lifespan –of course, granted that God does not decide otherwise, accidents do not occur , and there are no "crazies" with unrestricted access to guns .

There are also other new medical inventions in progress; some are longevity-promoting drugs, formulated from resveratrol, a chemical derived from berries, like grapes (Walters, 2013) , and others are computerized gadgets that can video record dreams .

The claims that God lives within us are not frivolous. "Your body is the physical manifestation of the sum of your life's experiences...It is the outward reflection of your precious inner life." (Rankin, 2013) It symbolizes the complex operations of the unseen realm of the Creator God. The body's physiological constitution is the material representation of the unseen Spiritual world of God.

God is Trinity. He has created human beings as trichotomy. The brain is symbolic of God, complex, and always radiating its electrical energy as God is light; he is unfathomable, and there is no darkness in him. (1 John 1:5).

The heart is a symbol of Jesus Christ, the human face of God's love and compassion. The scripture describes Christ as "the visible image of the invisible God. " (1 Colossians 1:15) The lung is symbolic of the Holy Spirit. Genesis states that " the LORD God ... breathed into (human) his nostrils the breath of life, and the man became a living being." (Genesis 2:7) The brain, heart and lung , the three as trichotomy in one human body, operate in synchrony, as God the Father God the Son God the Holy Spirit, the Holy Trinity is One.

God wants us to live a long life. He will reward those who love and obey him, "with long life and show them his salvation." (Psalm 91: 14-16) Salvation is not for a future time after this life. Salvation does not begin only when Jesus comes again. God's salvation is here and now for those who love and obey him. "There is severe discipline for one who forsakes the way, but the one who hates rebukes will die." (Proverbs 15:10) The disobedient world is facing God's wrath! God warned ,

> I will destine you to the sword , and all of you shall bow down to the slaughter; because when I called, you did not answer, but when I spoke, you did not listen, but you did what was evil in my sight, and chose what I did not delight in. (Isaiah 65:12).

Those that obey God and give themselves to his Son Jesus, have their eternal salvation. They will "flourish like palm trees and grow strong like the cedars." (Psalm 92:12) They will live to be 120 years and beyond.

If you have wandered off far away from Jehovah, please repent and come back home to your Father. Jehovah God will forgive your sins; "all of us have sinned , and have come short of the glory of God."

(Romans 3:23) It is not too late to call on Jesus to save you. Pray for forgiveness.

Are you a backslider ? Do not die unrepentant. Look to Jesus. He is in the Father. Together, the Father, Son and the Holy Spirit say, , "If my people, who are called by my name, will humble themselves and pray and seek my face and turn from their wicked ways, then I will hear from heaven, and I will forgive their sin and will heal their land." (2 Chronicles 7:14) And you, non-believer, do not perish in your unbelief. Jehovah God takes " no pleasure in the death of the wicked, but rather that they turn from their ways and live. Turn! Turn from your evil ways! Why will you die...? (Ezekiel 33:11)

You do not know if you would be dead within the next few minutes or days. Eternity in hell is a very, long time , so please , "seek the Lord while he may be found; call on him while he is near. " (Isaiah 55:6)

Repent, and return to the Lord. Please say a prayer along these lines ; "Father Almighty, Omnipotent, Omniscient God, Pantocrator; the Maker of heaven and earth, I am here with a contrite heart, feeling very sorry for my sins. Father God, there's nothing that can wash away my sins but by the blood of your only Son my Lord Jesus Christ. I believe He was conceived by the Holy Spirit, born of the virgin Mary. He was crucified and he died for my sins so that my sins will be forgiven. He rose again the third day,and ascended to heaven where He is sitting on your right side interceding for my sins all the time.

I believe He will come back again, to judge the living and the dead. I believe in the resurrection of the dead. I believe your Holy Spirit is working in me, cleansing me, changing me, sanctifying me, justifying me, and saving me.

I thank you O Jehovah God for forgiving my sins. Lord Jesus Christ, I thank you for giving your life away for my salvation. I believe you died for me. I repent my sins. Please make me yours. Make me whole. Now I know I am free from Satan's bondage.

Holy Spirit, come, and dwell in me. Guide me. Direct my path. Help me to live like Christ Jesus. I give you thanks, I give you the glory, Almighty Father. I pray in Jesus name. Amen. I'm saved. I'm delivered. Praise the LORD. Find yourself a bible teaching, God – loving, Christ believing church, or contact us by email biblicalhealthcenter@gmail.com   twitter.com/biblicalh or by mail

Biblical Health Center Inc Nonprofit

P.O.Box 291964

Tampa, Fl 33687

The Author.

First, I did not think I needed to make any
statement about me because this book is not about
myself. I believe that Jehovah God is only using me to
deliver his message since it is not impossible for God to
raise a stone to speak for him . Once he caused a
donkey to speak so why would he not raise a stone to
speak if he so desired? Did Jehovah not make Adam out
of dust? But when I reflected on a teaching by our Lord
Jesus which reminds us "there will be more rejoicing in
heaven over one sinner who repents," (Luke 15:7) I
thought that by telling this story, I may help somebody
find his or her way back to Jesus ?

With this consideration, I make this declaration:
I am one hundred years old , with twenty-four more
years yet to go. I am working on my bachelor's degree
in Applied Science at Siena Heights University College
of Professional Studies, Adrian, Michigan. (It is
important that nobody thinks he or she is "too old to go
to College.")

Fourteen years ago, I moved to Tampa, Florida
from New York City, a very sick man. I was so sick that
my doctors expected me to die. When I moved to
Tampa, Florida, I remained unemployed because my ill-

health would not allow me to work so without any money in reserve to pay my rent, I became homeless.

According to my doctors, I suffered, "multi-organ complications." But I am thankful for a compassionate personal care physician, Dr. Jon E. Hemstreet at Tampa General Hospital. Despite a hopeless prognosis, Dr. Hemstreet continued to give me hope to live even though my body refused treatment, and conventional medical opinion was that I was dying.

It was at that point that I decided I had to speak to Jesus the Son of Jehovah God. For , after all, I did not make my life, and if my brain, heart, lungs, and indeed every member of my body, had a Creator called Jehovah, it was my decision-making time to seek his face. It was my decision-making time to yield myself totally to his control whether I lived or died. Instead of focusing on the pains convulsing the members of my body, I decided to drown my thoughts and mind in studying the bible. In studying the bible, I discovered Jehovah God's assurance that he is the God " that heals", and that "plants are there for food and healing." (Ezekiel 47:12)

I decided to take Jehovah God at his word; I prayed for his guidance that I might find which bible plants would heal my illnesses.By doing so I discovered more than one hundred and twenty plant names in the bible. I spent time in the library afterward researching their medicinal uses. If the doctors' prescribed medications were not helping me recover, it did not make any sense that I continued taking them. Instead, I needed to trust Jesus with whatever he planned for my life and decided also to pay attention to the foods I ate. My meal consisted mainly of the vegetables , fruits , berries and the nuts I read about in the bible. I told my doctor I was not going to take any more medicines.

Here is Dr. Hemstreet to tell my story from his perspective :

I remember well the first time I met Kwasi Hezekiah Scipio . He had been discharged from the hospital and presented to my office very ill. His symptoms involved almost every system in his body. Because of his multi-organ involvement, his prognosis was quite poor although no definite diagnosis could be established in the hospital. Mr. Scipio and I discussed the next treatment steps we should take including additional testing, medications, and specialist consultation. Despite these further evaluations and more testing, his diagnosis remained elusive, and his condition did not improve. Mr. Scipio stated on one follow-up visit that he wanted to be withdrawn from some of his medications and that he would pursue natural healing methods. Initially, I was not in favor of this approach, but eventually we agreed to keep him only on essential medications and monitor his progress with natural remedies. Remarkably, with time, Mr. Scipio's condition improved to the point where his vital signs and laboratory values returned to normal... I am trained in western allopathic medicine and do not have expertise in natural remedies. In fact, I am sometimes skeptical of these treatments and was not enthusiastic, in the case of Mr. Scipio, to exchange his western medicine for natural ones. But his improvement has been a wonderful lesson for me in the power of natural substances to heal... Mr. Scipio has taught me other valuable lessons as well; his faith was not shaken. I also learned from Mr. Scipio the power of positive thinking. (Hemstreet , J (2006) Amazing Bible Healing Plants, Remedies and Recipes)

I took Jehovah God at his word, and focused on studying the bible as though the bible was a special letter from my father. I received miraculous gifts of recovery. I also received insights into things I did not know before. Jehovah God has forgiven my sins, and healed my diseases; he will satisfy me with good as long as I live so that my youth is renewed like eagle's .(Psalm 103:3-5)

He has allowed me to do things beyond my own natural abilities. Jehovah God has kept me alive and will use me along with his chosen believers to help to build in Tampa a Biblical Health Center where believers and the sick together will assemble and live by Matthew

22:34-40 , and where we will live and enjoy the goodness and mercy of Jehovah God.

A scoffer seeks wisdom in vain, but knowledge is easy for one who understands. Leave the presence of a fool, for there you do not find words of knowledge." (Proverbs 14:6-7)

References

Adventists health studies (n.d), Loma Linda University School of Public Health website. Retrieved from http://www.llu.edu/public-health/health/index.page

American Institute of Stress (2014), website. Retrieved from http://www.stress.org/daily-life/

Benson, H (n.d), Timeless healing. Video interview. Retrieved from https://www.youtube.com/watch?v=EOFbr-mf01Y

Fuhrman, (2005), Disease-proof your child, *Asthma and Allergies*, p.62-p70, St. Martin's Griffin, 175 Fifth Avenue, New York, N.Y. 10010.

Fuhrman, J (1995), Fasting and eating for health: a medical doctor's program for conquering disease. Retrieved from http://www.worldcat.org/title/fasting-and-eating-for-health-a-medical-doctors-program-for-conquering-disease/oclc/32311744&referer=brief_results

Harrington, A (2014) Church attendance is correlated with increased longevity. National Center for Complementary and Alternative Medicine video lecture . Retrieved from http://nccam.nih.gov/training/videolectures/8/2

Murphy P (2010, Feb 24) belief in a concerned God. Retrieved from

http://www.sciencedaily.com/releases/2010/02/100223132021.htm

New England journal of medicine (2005, Mar 17) a potential decline in life expectancy in the United States. Retrieved from http://www.nejm.org/doi/full/10.1056/nejmsr043743#t=article

Pappas, S (2013, Jan 20) Loneliness is bad for your health, study suggests . Retrieved from http://www.livescience.com/26431-loneliness-harms-health-immune-system.html

Pew Research (2013, Aug 8) Living to be 120 and beyond. Retrieved from *http://www.pewforum.org/2013/08/06/living-to-120-and-beyond-*

americans-views-on-aging-medical-advances-and-radical-life-extension/

Rosmarin D (2013) Faith in God positively influences treatment for individuals with psychiatric illnesses, website. Retrieved from http://www.sciencedaily.com/releases/2013/04/130425091606.htm

Saletan W (2013) Fear of immortality . Slate website. Retrieved fromhttp://www.slate.com/articles/technology/future_tense/2013/08/a ging_polls_and_life_extension_why_don_t_americans_want_to_live_ longer.html

Society for personality & social psychology (2013) Loneliness is bad for your health, study suggests. Website. Retrieved from http://www.livescience.com/26431-loneliness-harms-health-immune-system.html

Stangherlin M (2009) *The chiropractic way to health --   the ultimate self-help guide for chiropractic patients.* Indialantic Publishing, 1291-M Folly Road, Charleston, South Carolina 29412"

Walter, B (2013) Barbara Walters special | live to be 150. Video presentation. Retrieved from *https://www.youtube.com/watch?v=3CULtuGF1Xg*

Witvliet C van, Ludwig T. E & Laan, V.K. L (2001)."Granting forgiveness or harboring grudges". Research article. Retrieved from http://data.psych.udel.edu/rsimons/PSYC467/Witvliet%20et%20al.,% 202001.pdf

Worthington, E (1990) "The power of forgiveness", website. Retrieved from http://www.thepowerofforgiveness.com/about/peopleinthefilm/worthi ngton.html

www.ingramcontent.com/pod-product-compliance
Lightning Source LLC
Chambersburg PA
CBHW050338290526
45785CB00006B/2543